Metabolic Confusion for Beginners and Fast Weight Loss

Unlock Your Body's Fat Burning Potential With A Guide Featuring Mouthwatering Recipes, Meal Plan & Exercises to Boost Your Overall Health

Vince Cruise Sant

"Unlock Your Best Self: A Comprehensive Guide to Weight Loss and Wellness—From Nutrition to Metabolic Confusion, Celebrate Your Achievements on the Journey to Long-Term Success."

ABOUT THE AUTHOR

Introducing Vince Cruise Sant, a seasoned nutritionist with over a decade of dedicated experience in transforming lives through the power of balanced nutrition. With an extensive background in the field, Vince has emerged as a respected figure, dedicated to guiding individuals toward achieving their health and wellness aspirations.

With a wealth of practical knowledge and a deep understanding of nutrition and metabolism, Vince's expertise extends beyond theory. Having positively impacted the lives of more than 300 individuals, he stands as a testament to the tangible results his guidance brings.

Vince's approach transcends the conventional, recognizing the individuality of each person's journey toward well-being. His methodology seamlessly blends scientific insights with real-world application, ensuring that his advice is not only attainable but also sustainable.

Recognized as a trusted advisor and advocate for balanced nutrition, Vince Cruise Sant's commitment to empowering individuals is unwavering. His reputation as a compassionate and knowledgeable guide underscores his dedication to helping others unlock their full potential.

Whether you're a newcomer to the path of wellness or seeking to refine your existing practices, Vince's expertise will inspire and educate. Prepare to embark on a transformative journey led by a visionary who firmly believes that vibrant health is an achievable reality. With Vince's guidance, your pursuit of lasting well-being is poised for exceptional success.

TABLE OF CONTENTS

INTRODUCTION

There is a less-traveled path that transcends the ordinary and offers a revolutionary solution to the age-old struggle with excess weight. In a world where the pursuit of health and fitness has become an ever-elusive quest and where fad diets and miracle pills promise quick fixes but frequently lead to disappointment, This path is known as "metabolic confusion," and it has the ability to drastically alter your life, health, and body.

You've probably started your own personal path toward weight loss and a healthy lifestyle if you're reading this introduction. Maybe you've tried a ton of diets and workout plans, only to get stuck in a cycle of disappointment and resentment. We can relate to your difficulty, but we want to reassure you that there is an alternative that doesn't entail starving, restriction, or unsustainable exercise routines.

Metabolic confusion is not merely another fad in eating habits. It's a weight loss strategy that has changed the lives of countless people all over the world, is supported by science, has been tried and true, and is surprisingly effective. This book is a thorough guide to using metabolic confusion for rapid and long-lasting weight loss, whether you're a seasoned health enthusiast or just starting out on the path to a healthy you.

Why should you bother about metabolic confusion, and what exactly is it? Metabolic confusion is fundamentally a method of tricking your body. It puts pressure on your metabolism to adjust and function more effectively, which ultimately promotes better fat burning, greater energy, and overall better health. Metabolic confusion encourages you to embrace diversity, flexibility, and a greater awareness of your body's particular needs, in contrast to conventional diets that compel you to follow rigid routines.

We'll take you on a life-changing adventure through the world of metabolic confusion in this book. You will discover how to rewire your metabolism, escape the grip of unyielding fat, and live the active, healthy life you deserve. We'll provide you with step-by-step instructions that are both practical and scientifically sound, clarify the science underlying metabolic confusion, and arm you with the information you need to make wise decisions about your diet, exercise routine, and lifestyle.

It's not just another weight reduction book; Metabolic Confusion for Beginners and Fast Weight Reduction are your ticket to a long, happy life. You will learn the following through the pages that follow:

The mechanisms via which metabolic confusion alters your body

- Methods for incorporating metabolic confusion into your day-to-day existence
- Nutritional knowledge that will guide you're eating decisions
- Exercise techniques that maximize fitness gains and fat loss
- Reliable techniques for monitoring your development and maintaining motivation
- Ways to get beyond common weight reduction roadblocks and plateaus
- A plan for accomplishing your weight loss objectives and maintaining success over the long run

Metabolic Confusion for Beginners and Fast Weight Loss is your success manual, whether you have battled weight issues for years or are just starting your path to improved health. So that you can restore control over your body, improve your health, and finally achieve the rapid and long-lasting weight loss you've been hoping for, join us as we explore the secrets of metabolic confusion.

Are you prepared to start this trip that will change your life? The journey to a happier, healthier self-starts right now.

CHAPTER ONE

GETTING STARTED

Assessing Your Current Lifestyle

If you want to alter your life for the better, especially if you want to lose weight or adopt a healthier lifestyle, you must first evaluate your existing way of life. Your everyday habits, rituals, and decisions are all included in your lifestyle, which has a big impact on your general health and happiness.

1. Physical Activity: Workout Routine: Consider your present workout routine. What kinds of exercises do you love doing, and how frequently do you exercise?

Sedentary Behavior: Calculate how much of your day is spent sitting down or being inactive, such as watching TV or working at a desk.

2. Dietary routines: Examine your everyday eating patterns and routines. How frequently do you eat, and what kinds of foods make up your typical meals?

Portion Sizes: Consider your dietary intake. Do you typically eat too much or too little? Do you practice portion control?

2. Food Selections: Think about the caliber of the foods you select. How frequently do you eat fast food, processed meals, or sugary snacks?

Hydration: Consider how much water you consume. Do you regularly consume enough water throughout the day, or do you like sugary or caffeinated drinks more?

3. Sleeping Patterns: Sleep Duration: Calculate the average amount of sleep you receive each night. Do you regularly get adequate, restful sleep?

Sleeping Conditions: Consider the caliber of your sleep. Do you struggle to get to sleep or stay asleep? Are you rested when you wake up?

4. Stress Management:

Stressors: Determine the primary ongoing and situational sources of stress in your life. These can concern your job, your relationships, or other aspects of your life.

Coping strategies: Evaluate your stress management skills. Do you have healthy strategies for managing stress, or do you resort to unhealthy habits like overeating or excessive drinking?

5. Social and Emotional Well-Being:

Social Connections: Consider the strength of your social relationships. How often do you connect with friends and loved ones?

Emotional Health: Reflect on your emotional state. Are you generally happy and content, or do you frequently experience negative emotions like anxiety or sadness?

6. Medical History and Health Conditions:

Medical History: Review your medical history and any pre-existing health conditions. Are there any specific health concerns or medications you need to consider in your lifestyle assessment?

7. Habits and Addictions:

Smoking and Alcohol: If applicable, assess whether you smoke or consume alcohol and in what quantities.

Other Habits: Consider any other habits or addictions that may impact your health, such as excessive caffeine intake or recreational drug use.

8. Time Management:

Daily Schedule: Analyze how you allocate your time each day. Are you effectively balancing work, leisure, and personal time?

9. Environmental Factors:

Home and Work Environment: Evaluate your home and work environments for factors that could influence your lifestyle, such as access to healthy foods, exercise equipment, or opportunities for physical activity.

10. Health Goals and Values:

Personal Goals: Define your health and wellness goals. What do you want to achieve with your lifestyle changes, and why are these goals important to you?

Setting Realistic Goals

Any road toward self-improvement, including quick weight loss through metabolic confusion, starts with setting reasonable goals. Because they keep you motivated, allow you to monitor your progress, and give you a sense of accomplishment, realistic goals are crucial.

1. Be particular: Make a list of your objectives. Having a general goal like "lose weight" is less beneficial than having specific ones like "lose 10 pounds in two months" or "exercise for 30 minutes five days a week."

2. Make them measurable: Your objectives should be measurable so that you can keep tabs on your advancement. To gauge success, use figures or precise measurements. For instance, "run a 5k in under 30 minutes" or "reduce body fat percentage by 5%."

3. Set a timeframe: Assign your objectives a reasonable time frame. A deadline instills a sense of urgency and keeps you focused. I'll, for instance, "achieve my goal within three months" or "by the end of the year."

4. Consider Your Current Situation: Think about your lifestyle, level of exercise, and overall health right now. Consider your starting point while setting your objectives. Too aggressive goals should be avoided given your existing situation.

5. Break them down: If your long-term objective is substantial, divide it into smaller, easier-to-achieve goals. Your motivation will remain high as a result of reaching these objectives.

6. Make them achievable: Be realistic about your capabilities. Setting impossible ambitions might cause disillusionment and resentment. Determine your goals based on your skills, resources, and dedication.

7. Relevance: Make sure your objectives relate to your broader aims and values. Why are each of your goals significant to you? Ask yourself. You are more likely to be motivated to achieve goals that align with your values.

8. Specify both immediate and long-term objectives: Organize your goals into short-term (weeks or months) and long-term (several months to a year or more) categories. Long-term goals give you a bigger picture, while short-term goals keep you on track.

9. Prioritize your health and safety: Prioritize your health and safety by concentrating on objectives that advance your wellbeing. Avoid setting extreme goals that could endanger your wellbeing.

10. Seek Professional Guidance: If you have certain health issues or conditions, go to a doctor or a trained fitness professional who can help you set realistic goals.

11. Be flexible: Be ready to change your goals if necessary. The course of life is not always predictable, and things might alter. The secret to long-term success is adaptability.

12. Visualize Success: Picture yourself accomplishing your objectives. You can increase your motivation and maintain your commitment to your goals by using visualization.

13. Write them down: Write down your objectives in a journal or on a vision board: Writing them down strengthens your commitment and makes them more real.

14. Share Them: Take into account telling a family member or close friend about your objectives so they can encourage you and hold you accountable.

15. Track Your Progress: Evaluate your progress toward your objectives on a regular basis. To maintain accountability, use monitoring apps, photographs, or journal entries.

Creating a Weight Loss Plan

When using metabolic confusion tactics, having a solid weight loss plan in place is very important for reaching your objectives.

1. **Establish Specific Goals:**
   - Specify your desired weight loss goals, including how much weight you want to reduce and when you want to do it. Make sure your objectives are attainable and practical.

2. Determine Your Caloric Requirements:

- Depending on your age, gender, weight, height, and degree of exercise, determine your daily calorie requirements. For a more precise calculation, you can utilize internet calculators or speak with a trained nutritionist.

3. Pick Your Metabolic Confusion Techniques:

- Decide which metabolic confusion strategies you wish to use in your strategy. HIIT, calorie cycling, intermittent fasting, and carb cycling are a few examples of possible techniques in this category.

4. Establish a Meal Plan:

- Create a healthy food plan that reflects your calorie requirements and metabolic confusion techniques. Give whole foods like lean proteins, fresh produce, whole grains, and healthy fats top priority.

- Make sure you get a variety of macronutrients (proteins, carbs, and fats) in your meals and snacks throughout the day to maintain your energy levels and satiety.

- If you choose to engage in intermittent fasting, take into account when to eat and when to snack.

19

5. Plan a workout that combines both aerobic and weight training:

- **Plan Your Exercise Schedule:** Create a workout schedule. To improve adherence, incorporate exercises you enjoy.
- Plan your workouts throughout the week, aiming for the minimum amount of moderate-intensity aerobic exercise (150 minutes) or vigorous-intensity aerobic exercise (75 minutes) per week as advised by health standards.
- Include resistance training and HIIT sessions to increase metabolism and encourage muscular building.

6. Set a weekly schedule:

- For your activities, taking into account things like employment, family obligations, and personal preferences.
- Schedule time for meal preparation, physical activity, and downtime to maintain a balanced lifestyle.

7. Track your progress:

- Keep a notebook to keep track of your daily dietary intake, exercise routines, and any changes in your weight and other physical characteristics.
- Use tracking applications or wearable fitness equipment to keep an eye on your heart rate, steps taken, and calories burned.

8. Maintain Hydration:

- Make sure you get enough water to drink throughout the day. Dehydration can occasionally be mistaken for hunger, which encourages pointless nibbling.

9. Prepare for Challenges:

- Identify potential roadblocks and devise plans of action to get through them. This might entail overcoming urges, controlling stress, or avoiding harmful foods.

10. Seek Support:

- Share your weight loss plan and objectives with a sympathetic friend or relative. It might be quite helpful to have someone to motivate and inspire you.

11. Regularly Review and Adjust:

- Regularly evaluate your progress and make any plan modifications. Be ready for plateaus and setbacks because weight loss is not always consistent and progressive.

12. Consult a Professional:

- If you have underlying medical issues or special dietary needs, you may want to get tailored advice from a registered dietitian or other healthcare professional.

Importance of Consulting a Healthcare Professional

When starting any weight reduction or health improvement journey, even when adopting metabolic confusion strategies, consulting a healthcare expert is of the utmost importance.

1. Safety First: Medical professionals, including doctors, registered dietitians, and fitness specialists, can evaluate your present state of health and make tailored suggestions that put your safety first. They can spot any underlying illnesses or contraindications that can affect your attempts to lose weight.

2. Individualized Guidance: Everybody's body is different, so what works well for one person might not function well for another. A weight loss program can be specially created for you by healthcare professionals, taking into account your medical history, genetics, lifestyle, and preferences.

3. Addressing Underlying Health Issues: Health concerns including thyroid problems, diabetes, and hormonal imbalances can have an impact on metabolism and weight. These disorders can be identified and treated by a healthcare professional, who will also make sure they don't impede your development.

4. Medication Assessment: If you're currently taking medication, a medical expert can determine whether it might have an effect on your attempts to lose weight. If required, they can modify your prescription schedule or offer advice on how to deal with probable adverse effects.

5. Nutritional Guidance: Registered dietitians are nutrition specialists who can assist you in developing a balanced meal plan that supports your weight loss objectives and satisfies your nutritional requirements. Additionally, they can address particular dietary issues or constraints.

6. Behavioral Support: Medical specialists can offer insightful information on the psychological components of weight loss, such as emotional eating, stress reduction, and behavior modification. They can provide you with tactics for overcoming challenges and forming better habits.

7. Tracking Progress: Regular check-ins with a medical expert provide continuing progress tracking. They can monitor alterations in weight, body composition, and other health markers and make corrections as necessary.

8. Preventing nutritional deficits: Extreme weight reduction techniques and crash diets might result in nutrient deficits. By ensuring you maintain a balanced and nutrient-rich diet, healthcare professionals can assist you in avoiding these dangers.

9. Long-Term Success: Weight loss involves more than just losing weight; it also entails developing and sustaining a healthy lifestyle. Experts in medicine can advise you on how to maintain your results over the long run and avoid gaining weight.

10. Accountability and Support: Having a medical professional by your side as a supportive companion can help you stay motivated, hold yourself accountable, and get encouragement. Your devotion and self-assurance may increase when you are aware that you have someone to turn to for advice.

11. Evidence-Based Approaches: Medical experts base their recommendations on scientific research and evidence-based procedures. In the crowded world of weight reduction advice, they can assist you in separating fact from myth.

12. Holistic Approach: Healthcare practitioners frequently adopt a holistic perspective on health, addressing both weight loss and general well-being. They can assist you in shifting your attention from the scale to enhancing your overall health.

7-Day Meal Plan for those getting started with the Metabolic Confusion for Beginners and Fast Weight Loss

Day 1: Low-Carb Day

Breakfast: Scrambled eggs with spinach and tomatoes.

Snack: Greek yogurt with berries.

Lunch: Grilled chicken breast with a side salad (lettuce, cucumbers, bell peppers, and vinaigrette dressing).

Snack: Almonds or walnuts.

Dinner: Baked salmon with steamed broccoli and quinoa

Day 2: High-Carb Day

Breakfast: oatmeal topped with sliced banana and a sprinkle of cinnamon.

Snack: Apple slices with almond butter.

Lunch: Turkey and avocado wrap with whole-grain tortilla

Snack: carrot sticks with hummus.

Dinner: brown rice with stir-fried tofu and mixed vegetables.

Day 3: Medium-Carb Day

Breakfast: Smoothie with spinach, banana, protein powder, and almond milk

Snack: Cottage cheese with pineapple.

Lunch: Quinoa salad with chickpeas, cherry tomatoes, and feta cheese.

Snack: mixed nuts.

Dinner: Grilled shrimp with asparagus and a sweet potato

Day 4: Low-Carb Day

Breakfast: frittata with mushrooms, bell peppers, and cheese.

Snack: Sliced cucumber with cream cheese.

Lunch: Salad with grilled steak, mixed greens, and balsamic vinaigrette

Snack: cherry tomatoes with mozzarella cheese.

Dinner: Baked chicken breast with roasted Brussels sprouts and cauliflower mash.

Day 5: High-Carb Day

Breakfast: whole-grain toast with avocado and poached eggs.

Snack: strawberries with cottage cheese.

Lunch: lentil soup with a side of whole-grain crackers.

Snack: Edamame beans.

Dinner: Baked cod with quinoa and steamed broccoli

Day 6: Medium-Carb Day

Breakfast: Greek yogurt parfait with granola and mixed berries

Snack: Sliced bell peppers with hummus.

Lunch: Turkey and vegetable stir-fry with brown rice

Snack: mixed nuts and dried fruits.

Dinner: Grilled chicken with quinoa and steamed green beans.

Day 7: Low-Carb Day

Breakfast: spinach and feta omelet

Snack: celery sticks with peanut butter.

Lunch: tuna salad with mixed greens and vinaigrette dressing.

Snack: hard-boiled eggs.

Dinner: Baked tilapia with asparagus and mashed cauliflower

CHAPTER TWO

NUTRITION BASICS

The Role of Nutrition in Weight Loss

Weight loss is fundamentally influenced by nutrition. In addition to affecting your calorie intake, it also has an impact on your metabolism, hormones, and general wellness.

1. Caloric Deficit: You must consume fewer calories than you expend in order to lose weight. As a result, there is a calorie deficit, which forces your body to burn fat reserves for energy. To lose weight, one must create a calorie deficit that is healthy and sustained.

2. Macronutrient Balance: The proportions of the macronutrients you eat—carbohydrates, proteins, and fats—can affect your ability to lose weight. You may feel full longer, keep your muscles in shape, and improve your general health with a balanced diet that contains these macronutrients in the right amounts.

3. Protein: Protein helps maintain muscle mass, speeds up metabolism, and encourages feelings of fullness, all of which are essential for weight loss. It is advantageous to include lean protein sources in your diet, such as chicken, fish, tofu, and lentils.

4. Carbohydrates: Despite the promotion of low-carb diets for weight loss, carbohydrates are a vital source of energy. Choose complex carbs, which offer fiber and sustained energy, such as whole grains, fruits, and vegetables.

5. Fats: Healthy fats are necessary for satiety and nutritional absorption. Examples of these fats are those in avocados, almonds, and olive oil. They should be moderately incorporated into your diet.

6. Fiber: Consuming fewer calories overall is made possible by foods high in fiber, such as whole grains, fruits, and vegetables.

7. Hydration: Maintaining a healthy level of hydration is essential for weight loss. Sometimes hunger and thirst are confused. Before meals, drinking water can help you manage your hunger.

8. Meal Timing: Meal and snack times can affect weight loss. Smaller, more frequent meals that are balanced will help you manage your hunger and avoid overeating.

9. Mindful Eating: Keeping an eye on your food and eating habits will help you avoid mindless snacking and overeating. Eat without interruption and pay attention to your body's signals of hunger and fullness.

10. Portion Control: Pay attention to serving sizes. Even nutritious meals might cause weight gain if they are consumed in excess.

11. Nutrient-Dense Meals: Pay attention to meals that are high in nutrients and low in calories while still supplying necessary vitamins and minerals. These foods aid in both weight loss and general wellness.

12. Avoid sugary and processed foods: high-sugar and highly processed foods may cause overeating and weight gain. Reduce their consumption.

13. Individualization: Each person has unique nutritional requirements. What is effective for one person might not be effective for another. In order to create a customized nutrition plan, think about speaking with a registered dietitian or other healthcare expert.

14. Long-Term Lifestyle Change: When weight loss is part of a long-lasting lifestyle change, it is most effective. Extreme limitations and crash diets frequently don't work long-term and can cause weight gain.

Macronutrients and Micronutrients

Our bodies require two types of vital nutrients in order to function properly: macronutrients and micronutrients. The quantity needed and the functions they serve in preserving health vary.

Macronutrients

1. Quantity Required: The body needs macronutrients in significant amounts. The majority of your daily caloric intake comes from them.

2. Main Categories: There are three main classes into which macronutrients are divided:

- Carbohydrates: The body uses carbohydrates as its main source of energy. They consist of fibers, starches, and sugars.
- Proteins: Proteins are necessary for the development and repair of tissues as well as for a number of metabolic activities.
- Fats (lipids): Fats are a second source of energy and are necessary for the absorption of vitamins that are fat-soluble as well as for insulation and organ protection.

3. Calories: Macronutrients give the body calories, or energy. In comparison to fat, which has roughly 9 calories per gram, carbohydrates and proteins have about 4 calories per gram.

4 Examples:

Carbohydrates: Bread, rice, pasta, fruits, vegetables.

Proteins: Meat, fish, eggs, dairy products, legumes, tofu.

Fats: Avocado, nuts, oils, butter, fatty fish.

5. Functions:

- Carbohydrates give you rapid energy for work-related tasks and physical activity.
- Proteins are necessary for the development, maintenance, and repair of tissues.
- Fats act as a long-lasting energy source, sustain cell structure, and offer cushioning for organs.

Micronutrients:

1. Quantity Required: Micronutrients are required in significantly lesser amounts than macronutrients. Usually, these are expressed as milligrams (mg) or micrograms (mcg).

2. Main Categories: There are two main categories for micronutrients:

Vitamins: organic substances necessary for a variety of metabolic functions, growth, and general health. Vitamins C, D, and the B complex are a few examples.

Minerals: inorganic nutrients needed for processes like maintaining fluid balance, neuron signaling, and bone health. Iron, zinc, and calcium are some examples.

3. **Calories:** Although micronutrients do not directly produce calories, they are essential to metabolic processes that allow the body to use macronutrients as fuel.

4. **Examples:**

- Vitamins, such as Vitamin K (found in leafy greens), Vitamin A (found in carrots), and Vitamin C (found in citrus fruits).
- **Minerals:** zinc (found in nuts and seeds), iron (found in red meat), and calcium (found in dairy products).

5. **Functions:**

- Vitamins and minerals are necessary for a number of biological processes, such as energy production, bone health, blood coagulation, and immune system support.

- Specific health issues like scurvy (vitamin C deficiency) or anemia (iron shortage) can be brought on by micronutrient deficits.

Understanding Calories

The amount of energy in the meals and beverages we consume is measured in calories. When we consume and metabolize these sources, they can provide our bodies with a certain quantity of energy.

The following key points can assist you in understanding calories:

1. Caloric Value: Calories, or "calories" for short, are commonly defined in terms of energy units called kilocalories (kcal). The energy required to raise the temperature of one gram of water by one degree Celsius is measured in calories (Cal). Typically, when we discuss calories in relation to food, we are referring to kilocalories.

2. Energy Balance: The ideas of calories and energy balance are intertwined. The calories you take in from food and drink should about match the calories you burn through activity, resting metabolic rate, and other biological processes to maintain your present weight. You gain weight if you eat more calories than you burn; you lose weight if you eat fewer calories.

3. Micronutrient Sources: Various macronutrients have varying calorie counts per gram, including:

- There are around 4 calories per gram of carbohydrates.
- About 4 calories are contained in each gram of protein.
- There are roughly 9 calories per gram of fat (lipids).
- **Alcohol:** Although it is not a macronutrient, it contains about 7 calories per gram and increases calorie consumption.

4. Basic Metabolic Rate (BMR): Your BMR is the amount of energy your body requires to maintain fundamental processes like breathing, circulation, and cell formation while at rest. Individual differences exist and are influenced by things like age, gender, weight, and muscle mass.

5. Total Daily Energy Expenditure (TDEE): Taking into account your BMR and degree of physical activity, TDEE is the total number of calories your body requires each day. It is essential to figure out how many calories you need to eat in order to gain, maintain, or decrease weight.

6. Weight management: To lose weight, you must consume fewer calories than your body uses up in a 24-hour period. You must consume more calories than you burn in order to produce a calorie surplus and gain weight. Your calorie intake and expenditure must be equal if you want to maintain your weight.

7. Nutrient Quality: While calorie intake is crucial for weight management, so is the caloric quality of those calories. Those that are high in nutrients also contain significant amounts of vital vitamins, minerals, and other health-promoting components, as opposed to those that are high in calories but nothing else (such as sugary snacks).

8. Dietary Guidelines: National health organizations offer dietary recommendations that specify calorie limits depending on factors like age, gender, and degree of activity. These tips are meant to be general ones for being healthy.

9. Calorie Tracking: Some people decide to monitor their calorie consumption with the aid of devices like food diaries or mobile applications. This can help you manage your weight, but you should use caution to maintain a balanced diet.

Building a Balanced Diet

Building a balanced diet is essential for maintaining good health and well-being. Here are 10 steps to help you create a well-rounded and nutritious eating plan:

1. Assess Your Goals: Determine your specific dietary goals, whether it's weight management, improving overall health, or meeting specific nutritional needs.

2. Understand Your Caloric Needs: Calculate your total daily energy expenditure (TDEE) to determine the number of calories you need each day to maintain your current weight. Adjust this number based on your goals (e.g., create a calorie deficit for weight loss or a surplus for weight gain).

3. Include a Variety of Food Groups: Aim to incorporate foods from all major food groups:

- Fruits
- Vegetables
- Grains (preferably whole grains)
- Lean proteins (e.g., poultry, fish, tofu, legumes)

- Dairy or dairy alternatives (e.g., yogurt, fortified plant-based milk)

4. Prioritize Vegetables: Make vegetables a significant part of your diet. They are rich in vitamins, minerals, fiber, and antioxidants. Aim to fill half your plate with vegetables at meals.

5. Choose Whole Grains: opt for whole grains over refined grains. Whole grains like brown rice, quinoa, and whole wheat pasta provide more nutrients and fiber.

6. Include lean proteins: Incorporate lean sources of protein into your diet to support muscle health and satiety while reducing saturated fat intake. Examples include skinless poultry, fish, beans, and tofu.

7. Monitor fat intake: Focus on healthy fats, such as those found in avocados, nuts, seeds, and olive oil. Limit saturated and trans fats found in fried foods, processed snacks, and fatty cuts of meat.

8. Control Portion Sizes: Be mindful of portion sizes to avoid overeating. Use smaller plates and pay attention to hunger and fullness cues.

9. Limit Added Sugars and Salt: Minimize the consumption of foods and beverages high in added sugars and sodium. Check food labels to identify hidden sources of these ingredients.

10. Stay Hydrated: Drink plenty of water throughout the day. Limit sugary drinks and excessive caffeine intake.

11. Plan balanced meals: Create balanced meals that include a protein source, a serving of vegetables or fruits, and a whole grain. This combination provides a variety of nutrients and helps keep you satisfied.

12. Snack wisely: Choose nutritious snacks like Greek yogurt, nuts, fruits, or cut-up vegetables with hummus to curb hunger between meals.

13. Practice mindful eating: pay attention to what you eat, savor each bite, and eat without distractions. This can help prevent overeating and promote a healthy relationship with food.

14. Moderation is Key: It's okay to enjoy occasional treats and indulgences, but do so in moderation.

15. Seek Professional Guidance: If you have specific dietary needs or health concerns, consider consulting a registered dietitian or healthcare professional for personalized guidance and meal planning.

CHAPTER THREE

METABOLIC CONFUSION TECHNIQUES

Cycling Calories

The feeding strategy known as "cycling calories" is frequently applied in the context of metabolic confusion techniques with the aim of fostering weight loss and metabolic adaptation. Using this method, you deliberately alter your daily calorie intake over a certain time period, usually in a cyclical fashion, in an effort to trigger a metabolic response that may promote fat loss and inhibit metabolic adaptation. Let's delve more into this idea.

The Function of Cycling Calories:

1. High-Calorie Days: You may purposefully consume more calories on some days than your typical maintenance amount. These days are frequently referred to as "high-calorie" or "re-feed" days. The intention is to temporarily increase your metabolism and give you more energy for exercise.

2. Low-Calorie Days: In contrast, you consume fewer calories on other days in order to generate a calorie deficit. These are frequently referred to as "fasting" or "low-calorie" days. The fewer calories you consume, the more your body is stimulated to burn off stored fat for energy, which helps you lose weight.

The aspect of metabolic confusion

The idea behind "metabolic confusion" is that you can possibly stop your metabolism from adjusting to a constant calorie deficit by alternating between days with high and low caloric intake. This is based on the theory that, over time, weight loss may become more difficult since your body may modify how much energy it expends in response to continuous calorie restriction.

Key advantages and things to think about

1. Preventing Plateaus: Altering your caloric intake can help you move past weight loss stalemates. Your body may react more strongly to changes in calorie consumption than it would if you were always in a calorie deficit.

2. Preserving Muscle: Cycling calories can help you maintain your muscle mass while you're losing weight since higher-calorie days give you enough protein and energy to keep your muscles healthy and strong.

3. Psychological Benefits: Because cycling calories allows for occasional higher-calorie meals or days, some people find it more manageable and durable than continuous calorie restriction.

4. Customization: Individual tastes and objectives can be taken into account when determining the frequency and intensity of calorie cycling. Some people might like a more moderate strategy, while others would want more notable calorie swings.

5. Potential Challenges: For some people, continuously implementing cycling calories may be difficult. It necessitates careful planning and tracking of daily caloric intake.

6. Nutrient Quality: For optimal health, it's important to select nutrient-dense foods regardless of calorie cycling. Constantly strive to eat a mix of fruits, veggies, lean proteins, and whole grains.

7. Consult a Professional: It is advised to speak with a trained dietitian or other healthcare provider before using any metabolic confusion or calorie cycling strategies. They can assist in adjusting the strategy to your unique needs and keep tabs on your development.

Intermittent Fasting

Cycling between times of eating and fasting is a key component of the popular dietary strategy known as intermittent fasting (IF). The purpose of this technique is to induce a controlled fasting state, which will optimize metabolic processes, enhance general health, and encourage weight loss. Let's explore intermittent fasting in greater detail.

Learning about Intermittent Fasting

The two primary periods of intermittent fasting are alternated between:

1. Feeding Window: You eat your daily calorie intake during this phase. Depending on the particular IF procedure you choose, this window could be anything from a few hours to a whole day.

2. Fasting Window: During this period, you restrict calorie intake to force your body to use its energy stores. The length of this fasting phase can also change based on the IF method used.

Typical Intermittent Fasting Techniques:

There are a number of well-known IF protocols, each with particular fasting and feeding windows:

1. The 16/8 Method: This entails a 16-hour fast each day and an 8-hour interval for eating. You might, for instance, eat from 12:00 to 8:00 and then refrain from eating until 12:00 the next day.

2. The 5:2 Method: Using this strategy, you eat normally five days a week and limit your calorie intake to roughly 500–600 calories on the other two days that aren't consecutive.

3. Alternate-Day Fasting: In this technique, you alternate between eating days and fasting days, during which you consume few calories or none at all.

4. The Warrior Diet: This plan calls for a 20-hour fast followed by a 4-hour window of eating in the evening.

The aspect of metabolic confusion

Because it alters calorie intake and meal times, intermittent fasting might be viewed as a type of metabolic confusion. It puts your body's metabolic processes to the test by alternating between eating and fasting intervals, which may help prevent metabolic adaptation to a continuously low-calorie diet. Over time, this might help sustain a stable weight decrease.

Benefits and Things to Think About

1. **Weight Management:** Since IF naturally lowers calorie intake and promotes the body to burn stored fat for energy during fasting periods, it can be a useful tool for weight loss.

2. **Insulin Sensitivity:** IF might enhance insulin sensitivity, assisting in blood sugar regulation and lowering the risk of type 2 diabetes.

3. **Cellular Repair:** When you fast, your body starts cellular repair procedures, including autophagy, which can increase your lifespan and general wellness.

4. **Simplicity:** Since IF doesn't include intricate meal planning or calorie counting, it can be rather simple to follow.

5. **Individual Variation:** Depending on the user, IF may or may not be successful. It might work for some people's goals and lifestyles, but not for others.

6. **Hydration and Nutrient Quality:** It's essential for general health to stay hydrated and concentrate on nutrient-dense foods during the feeding window.

7. **Consultation:** Before beginning an intermittent fasting program, it is advised to speak with a healthcare provider

or trained dietitian, especially if you have underlying medical issues or dietary restrictions.

Carb Cycling

A dietary plan and metabolic confusion technique called carb cycling entails altering carbohydrate consumption on several days of the week. By systematically managing carbohydrate consumption, this method aims to increase athletic performance, optimize metabolism, and aid in weight management. Let's look more closely at carb cycling.

How to Understand Carb Cycling

Carb cycling entails alternating between days with a higher intake of carbohydrates, often known as "high-carb days," and days with a lower intake of carbohydrates, also referred to as "low-carb days. A planned fluctuation in carbohydrate intake is intended to affect metabolic processes and accomplish particular fitness or health goals.

The aspect of metabolic confusion

Because carb cycling provides fluctuations in calorie sources and macronutrient ratios with a primary concentration on carbohydrates, it might be seen as a sort of metabolic confusion. This method puts the body's ability to adapt to changes in carbohydrate and calorie intake to the test by switching between days with high and low carbohydrate intakes. This may aid in avoiding plateaus and maintaining the progression of weight reduction or muscle building.

How Carb Cycling Operates

1. High-Carb Days: You consciously consume a higher proportion of carbohydrates on certain days. This helps replenish glycogen stores, which are crucial for athletic performance and muscle repair, and provides an energy boost for strenuous workouts.

2. Low-Carb Days: You consume fewer carbohydrates on low-carb days and make up the difference by consuming more protein and good fats. This may encourage fat reduction by encouraging the body to utilize stored fat for energy.

Common carb cycling strategies include:

1. Classic Carb Cycling: Depending on personal objectives and preferences, this method often entails rotating between high-carb and low-carb days every two to three days.

2. Targeted Carb Cycling: Using this strategy, you eat higher-carb meals or snacks before or after workouts to aid in performance and recovery while consuming fewer carbohydrates on rest days.

3. Weekly Carb Cycling: Some people prefer a more regimented strategy, cycling carbohydrates on particular days of the week, such as high-carb days on training days when you work out hard and low-carb days on days when you rest or exercise less.

Benefits and Things to Think About

1. Optimized Performance: By supplying a carbohydrate boost when necessary while still allowing for fat utilization during low-carb phases, carb cycling can improve athletic performance.

2. Weight Management: When paired with a proper overall calorie intake, it can be a successful technique for both weight loss and muscle building.

3. Metabolic Adaptation: By preventing metabolic adaptation to ongoing low-carb diets, carb cycling may aid in long-term weight management.

4. Individual Variation: Different people respond differently to carb cycling. While some people react well, others might not see any real advantages.

5. Nutrient Quality: Prioritizing nutrient-dense sources of carbs, proteins, and fats will help you achieve your micronutrient demands while carb cycling.

6. Consultation: If you're thinking about carb cycling, talking to a certified dietitian or fitness expert can help you design a personalized strategy that fits your objectives and dietary preferences.

High-Intensity Interval Training (HIIT)

When carefully employed to enhance metabolic processes, promote fitness, and manage weight, high-intensity interval training (HIIT) is a well-liked workout approach that can be thought of as a metabolic confusion technique. Short bursts of intensive exercise are interspersed with rest or lower-intensity exercise during HIIT. This strategy puts the body's capacity for metabolic adaptation to the test, which could result in increased calorie burn and better metabolic health in general. Let's examine HIIT in more depth.

High-Intensity Interval Training (HIIT): An Overview

The intensity of HIIT and its alternating activity and rest periods are its defining features. Exercises like sprinting, cycling, leaping, or bodyweight exercises may be performed during a normal HIIT session at close to maximum effort for a brief amount of time (often 20 to 60 seconds), followed by a recovery or low-intensity period lasting roughly 10 to 30 seconds.

The aspect of metabolic confusion

Because HIIT introduces fluctuations in exercise intensity and duration, it can be viewed as a metabolic confusion approach. HIIT strains the body's energy systems by often alternating between high-intensity and recovery intervals, possibly preventing it from properly adjusting to one particular exercise intensity. This could result in a number of metabolic advantages.

How HIIT Operates:

1. Increased Calorie Burn: Exercise during and after HIIT increases heart rate and metabolism. Excess post-exercise oxygen consumption (EPOC), a phenomenon that occurs after exercise, refers to the body's continued calorie burning.

2. Fat Loss: HIIT, particularly during high-intensity intervals, might encourage the use of stored fat for energy, hence promoting fat loss.

3. Muscle Building: Although HIIT is largely renowned for its cardiovascular advantages, adding resistance workouts to the practice can also stimulate muscle growth and enhance muscular tone.

4. Cardiovascular Fitness: When compared to steady-state, moderate-intensity workouts, HIIT can increase cardiovascular endurance, oxygen uptake, and general fitness more quickly.

Typical HIIT protocols

1. Tabata: This well-known HIIT routine alternates 20 seconds of intense exercise with 10 seconds of rest for a total of 8 cycles in 4 minutes.

2. 1:1 Ratio: Using this technique, you alternate 1 minute of vigorous exercise with 1 minute of rest or light activity.

3. Pyramid: Pyramid HIIT sessions gradually lengthen the high-intensity intervals before shortening them again.

4. Fartlek Training: Fartlek, which translates to "speed play" in Swedish, is an unstructured variant of HIIT in which you adjust your workout's intensity and duration in accordance with how you feel.

Benefits and Things to Think About

1. Efficiency: While HIIT workouts are often shorter than steady-state workouts, they can nonetheless result in equivalent or better calorie burn and fitness gains.

2. Metabolic Boost: HIIT might result in a higher resting metabolic rate, which might enhance daily calorie expenditure.

3. Accessibility: HIIT is accessible to a wide range of people due to its adaptability to different fitness levels and preferences.

4. Variation: Preventing training monotony and plateaus by regularly switching up the routines, intervals, and intensity levels

5. Consultation: Before beginning an HIIT program, speak with a fitness expert or a medical professional, especially if you have existing health issues or are new to exercising.

Importance of Adequate Sleep

A key component of metabolic health is getting enough sleep, which can be used as a metabolic confusion strategy to improve overall wellbeing and optimize metabolic processes. Numerous metabolic processes, including hormone production, energy balance, and cellular repair, are significantly regulated by sleep. Let's examine the significance of getting enough sleep from a metabolic standpoint.

1. Regulation of hormones

The hormones that control appetite and hunger, in particular, need enough sleep to remain in a balanced hormonal state. Hormonal abnormalities caused by lack of sleep include:

Ghrelin: Lack of sleep can raise ghrelin levels, an appetite-stimulating hormone that heightens sensations of hunger.

Leptin: On the other hand, lack of sleep can cause leptin levels, a hormone that indicates fullness, to drop. As a result, satiety symptoms may be lessened.

Insulin: Insufficient sleep length and poor sleep quality can have a negative influence on insulin sensitivity, thereby raising the risk of type 2 diabetes and insulin resistance.

2. Energy regulation

The body's strategy for regulating its energy depends on sleep. A healthy amount of sleep aids in weight management by assisting the body in controlling how much energy it uses and expends. People who are sleep-deprived may feel:

- A rise in the desire for calorie-dense, sweet, and fatty meals.
- A decreased desire to exercise and engage in physical activities.
- Difficulty maintaining an active lifestyle due to increased fatigue and decreased overall energy levels

3. Cellular Maintenance and Repair:

For the body, sleep is a time of rest and restoration. Cellular repair and maintenance functions are increased during deep sleep periods. The elimination of waste products from cells, the growth and repair of tissues, and the release of growth hormone—all of which are crucial for general well-being and vitality—are included in this process.

4. Thermoregulation and Metabolic Rate:

The body's metabolism and thermoregulation are influenced by sleep. Lack of sleep can affect metabolic efficiency by lowering the basal metabolic rate (the amount of energy your body requires to function while at rest) and interfering with temperature regulation.

5. Stress management and cortisol control:

The management of stress and cortisol levels, a hormone produced in reaction to stress, depends on getting enough sleep. Chronic sleep loss can increase cortisol levels, which may encourage more fat to be stored, particularly around the abdomen.

6. Implications for Long-Term Health:

Numerous long-term health problems, including obesity, cardiovascular disease, hypertension, and a weakened immune system, have been related to chronic sleep deprivation. Additionally, it can have a severe effect on mental health, resulting in mood disorders including despair and anxiety.

7. Enhanced Cognitive Function

For cognitive function, memory consolidation, and decision-making, quality sleep is crucial. People who get enough sleep are better able to make wise dietary decisions and maintain a regular exercise regimen, both of which are crucial for metabolic health.

CHAPTER FOUR

MEAL PLANNING AND RECIPES

Weekly Meal Planning

Day 1: Monday

Breakfast:

- Scrambled eggs with spinach and tomatoes
- Whole-grain toast
- A serving of mixed berries

Lunch:

- Grilled chicken breast salad with mixed greens, cherry tomatoes, cucumbers, and balsamic vinaigrette dressing

Snack:

- Greek yogurt with honey and a sprinkle of nuts

Dinner:

- Baked salmon with lemon and dill
- Quinoa pilaf
- Steamed broccoli

Day 2: Tuesday

Breakfast:

- Oatmeal topped with sliced bananas and a dollop of almond butter

Lunch:

- Turkey and avocado wrap with whole-grain tortilla
- Side salad with a light vinaigrette

Snack:

- Carrot and cucumber stick with hummus

Dinner:

- Vegetarian chili with kidney beans, black beans, and plenty of veggies
- Brown rice.

Day 3: Wednesday

Breakfast:

- Greek yogurt parfait with granola and fresh berries

Lunch:

- Spinach and feta-stuffed chicken breast
- Quinoa salad with cucumber, red onion, and feta cheese

Snack:

- Apple slices with peanut butter

Dinner:

- Beef stir-fry with broccoli, bell peppers, and a ginger-soy sauce
- Steamed jasmine rice

Day 4: Thursday

Breakfast:

- Spinach and mushroom omelet
- Whole-grain toast

Lunch:

- Tuna salad with mixed greens, cherry tomatoes, and olives
- Whole-grain crackers

Snack:

- mixed nuts and dried fruits.

Dinner:

- Grilled shrimp skewers with a side of quinoa and roasted asparagus

Day 5: Friday

Breakfast:

- Smoothie with spinach, banana, Greek yogurt, and a spoonful of chia seeds

Lunch:

- Caprese salad with mozzarella cheese, tomatoes, and fresh basil
- whole-grain baguette.

Snack:

- Sliced bell peppers with hummus

Dinner:

- Baked chicken thighs with rosemary and garlic
- Mashed sweet potatoes
- Steamed green beans

Day 6: Saturday

Breakfast:

- Whole-grain pancakes with berries and a drizzle of maple syrup

Lunch:

- Lentil soup with a side of whole-grain bread

Snack:

- Cottage cheese with pineapple chunks

Dinner:

- Grilled tilapia with a mango salsa
- Quinoa and steamed broccoli

Day 7: Sunday

Breakfast:

- Veggie and cheese omelet
- whole-grain English muffin.

Lunch:

- Roast beef and Swiss cheese sandwich with whole-grain bread
- Side salad with your favorite dressing

Snack:

- A handful of grapes

Dinner:

- Vegetarian lasagna with layers of whole-grain pasta, spinach, mushrooms, and ricotta cheese
- A side of garlic bread

Sample Meal Plans

Day 1: High-Carb Day (Intermittent Fasting)

Breakfast:

- Scrambled eggs with spinach and tomatoes
- Whole-grain toast
- A serving of mixed berries

Lunch:

- Grilled chicken breast salad with mixed greens
- Cherry tomatoes
- Cucumbers
- Balsamic vinaigrette dressing
- A serving of quinoa or brown rice

Dinner:

- Baked salmon with lemon and dill
- Steamed broccoli
- Mashed sweet potatoes

Day 2: Low-Carb Day (Intermittent Fasting)

Breakfast:

- Greek yogurt parfait with granola and fresh strawberries

Lunch:

- Chickpea and vegetable stir-fry with a soy-ginger sauce
- Serve over brown rice or whole-grain noodles.

Dinner:

- Stuffed bell peppers with a mixture of quinoa, black beans, corn, and salsa
- Top with shredded cheese and bake until cheese is melted and bubbly.

Day 3: High-Carb Day (Intermittent Fasting)

Breakfast:

- Peanut butter and banana smoothie with a touch of honey

Lunch:

- Turkey and avocado wrap with whole-grain tortilla
- A side of mixed greens

Dinner:

- Shrimp scampi with garlic and lemon
- Serve over whole-grain pasta or zucchini noodles.

Day 4: Low-Carb Day (Intermittent Fasting)

Breakfast:

- Scrambled tofu with veggies and a sprinkle of sesame seeds

Lunch:

- Spinach and ricotta-stuffed pasta shells with marinara sauce

Dinner:

- Chicken or tofu curry with vegetables and coconut milk
- Serve over jasmine rice.

Day 5: High-Carb Day (Intermittent Fasting)

Breakfast:

- Caprese omelet with tomatoes, basil, and mozzarella cheese

Lunch:

- Greek salad with feta cheese, Kalamata olives, and a lemon-oregano vinaigrette
- Add grilled chicken or chickpeas for protein.

Dinner:

- Grilled lamb or eggplant kebabs with tzatziki sauce
- Serve with a side of tabbouleh (bulgur wheat salad).

Day 6: Low-Carb Day (Intermittent Fasting)

Breakfast:

- Labneh (strained yogurt) with olive oil, za'atar, and pita bread

Lunch:

- Falafel wrap with tahini sauce and a side of tabbouleh

Dinner:

- Beef or veggie fajitas with bell peppers and onions.
- Serve with brown rice and guacamole.

Day 7: High-Carb Day (Intermittent Fasting)

Breakfast:

- Banana and spinach smoothie with a scoop of protein powder

Lunch:

- Quinoa and black bean salad with a lime-cilantro dressing

Dinner:

- Grilled chicken breast with a side of sautéed spinach and quinoa

Day 8: Low-Carb Day (Intermittent Fasting)

Breakfast:

Scrambled eggs with sautéed mushrooms and a sprinkle of cheese

Lunch:

- Tuna salad with mixed greens, cherry tomatoes, and olives

Dinner:

- Baked cod or tofu with lemon and herbs
- Roasted Brussels sprouts

Day 9: High-Carb Day (Intermittent Fasting)

Breakfast:

- Blueberry and almond butter smoothie.

Lunch:

- Lentil soup with a side of whole-grain bread

Dinner:

- Teriyaki chicken or tofu with broccoli and brown rice

Day 10: Low-Carb Day (Intermittent Fasting)

Breakfast:

- Greek omelet with tomatoes, feta cheese, and olives

Lunch:

- Spinach and artichoke-stuffed chicken breasts
- Steamed asparagus

Dinner:

- Zucchini noodles with marinara sauce and meatballs or plant-based meatballs

Day 11: High-Carb Day (Intermittent Fasting)

Breakfast:

- Peanut butter and banana sandwich on whole-grain bread

Lunch:

- Roasted vegetable and quinoa bowl with tahini dressing

Dinner:

- Baked chicken with a side of sweet potatoes and green beans

Day 12: Low-Carb Day (Intermittent Fasting)

Breakfast:

- Scrambled eggs with diced bell peppers and onions

Lunch:

- Turkey and avocado lettuce wrap with a side of salsa

Dinner:

- Grilled shrimp with a side of asparagus and a Caesar salad

Day 13: High-Carb Day (Intermittent Fasting)

Breakfast:

- Overnight oats with almond milk, chia seeds, and mixed berries

Lunch:

- Caprese salad with mozzarella, tomatoes, basil, and balsamic glaze
- A serving of whole-grain crackers

Dinner:

- Stir-fried tofu or chicken with mixed vegetables and teriyaki sauce
- Serve over brown rice.

Day 14: Low-Carb Day (Intermittent Fasting)

Breakfast:

- Smoked salmon and cream cheese roll-ups

Lunch:

- Cabbage and ground beef stir-fry with a soy-ginger sauce

Dinner:

- Grilled steak or portobello mushrooms with a side of grilled zucchini and a garden salad

Delicious and Healthy Recipes

Breakfast

1. Greek Yogurt Parfait:

Ingredients:

- Greek yogurt
- Mixed berries
- Granola
- Honey

Instructions:

1. Layer Greek yogurt, mixed berries, and granola in a glass.
2. Drizzle with honey.
3. Enjoy!

2. Scrambled Eggs with Spinach:

Ingredients:

- Eggs
- Spinach
- Olive oil
- Salt and pepper

Instructions:

1. Heat olive oil in a pan, add spinach, and sauté until wilted.
2. Whisk the eggs, season with salt and pepper, and pour over the spinach.
3. Cook until the eggs are set, stirring occasionally.

3. Peanut Butter Banana Smoothie:

Ingredients:

- Banana
- Peanut butter
- Almond milk
- Greek yogurt
- Honey (optional)

Instructions:

1. Blend banana, peanut butter, almond milk, Greek yogurt, and honey until smooth.

4. Oatmeal with Berries:

Ingredients:

- Rolled oats
- Mixed berries
- Almond milk
- Honey (optional)

Instructions:

1. Cook oats with almond milk.

2. Top with mixed berries and a drizzle of honey.

5. Veggie Omelet:

Ingredients:

- Eggs
- Bell peppers
- Onions
- Tomatoes
- Spinach
- Olive oil
- Salt and pepper

Instructions:

1. Sauté bell peppers, onions, and tomatoes in olive oil.
2. Whisk the eggs, season with salt and pepper, and pour over the vegetables.
3. Cook until the eggs are set, folding the omelet in half.

6. Chia Pudding:

Ingredients: Chia seeds, Almond milk

- Vanilla extract
- Mixed berries

Instructions:

1. Mix chia seeds, almond milk, and a drop of vanilla extract.

2. Refrigerate overnight.

3. Top with mixed berries before serving.

7. Whole-Grain Pancakes:

Ingredients:

- Whole-grain pancake mix
- Fresh fruit (e.g., berries, sliced bananas)
- Greek yogurt

Instructions:

1. Prepare whole-grain pancakes as per the package instructions.

2. Top with fresh fruit and a dollop of Greek yogurt.

8. Avocado Toast:

Ingredients:

- Whole-grain toast
- Avocado
- Cherry tomatoes
- Red pepper flakes (optional)
- Salt and pepper

Instructions:

Mash avocado and spread it on toast.

Top with sliced cherry tomatoes and red pepper flakes (if desired), and season with salt and pepper.

9. Berry and Almond Butter Toast:

Ingredients:

- Whole-grain toast
- Almond butter
- Mixed berries
- Honey

Instructions:

1. Spread almond butter on toast.
2. Top with mixed berries and drizzle with honey.

10. Spinach and Mushroom Breakfast Quesadilla:

Ingredients: Whole-grain tortilla, Eggs, Spinach

- Mushrooms
- Cheese (optional)
- Olive oil
- Salt and pepper

Instructions:

1. Sauté spinach and mushrooms in olive oil.
2. Whisk eggs, season with salt and pepper, and scramble.

3. Place the egg mixture and cheese (if desired) on half of the tortilla and fold it in half.

4. Cook on a skillet until both sides are golden.

11. Blueberry Almond Butter Smoothie:

Ingredients:

- Blueberries
- Almond butter
- Almond milk
- Greek yogurt
- Honey (optional)

Instructions:

1. Blend blueberries, almond butter, almond milk, Greek yogurt, and honey until smooth.

12. Overnight Chia and Oat Pudding:

Ingredients:

- Chia seeds
- Rolled oats
- Almond milk
- Mixed berries

Instructions:

1. Mix chia seeds, rolled oats, and almond milk.

2. Refrigerate overnight.

3. Top with mixed berries before serving.

13. Sweet Potato Hash with Poached Eggs:

Ingredients:

- Sweet potatoes
- Bell peppers
- Onions
- Eggs
- Olive oil
- Paprika
- Salt and pepper

Instructions:

1. Sauté sweet potatoes, bell peppers, and onions in olive oil until tender.

2. Season with paprika, salt, and pepper.

3. Poach eggs and serve on top of the hash.

14. Green Smoothie Bowl:

Ingredients:

- Spinach
- Banana
- Pineapple

- Almond milk
- Toppings (e.g., granola, sliced almonds, chia seeds)

Instructions:

1. Blend spinach, banana, pineapple, and almond milk until smooth.
2. Pour into a bowl and add your favorite toppings.

15. Cottage Cheese and Fruit Bowl:

Ingredients:

- Cottage cheese
- Sliced peaches
- Almonds
- Honey

Instructions:

1. Top cottage cheese with sliced peaches, almonds, and a drizzle of honey.

Lunch
1. Grilled Chicken Salad:

Ingredients:

- Grilled chicken breast
- Mixed greens

- Cherry tomatoes
- Cucumbers
- Balsamic vinaigrette dressing

Instructions:

1. Slice grilled chicken breast and combine with mixed greens, cherry tomatoes, and cucumbers.
2. Drizzle with balsamic vinaigrette dressing.

2. Chickpea and Quinoa Bowl:

Ingredients:

- Cooked chickpeas
- Cooked quinoa
- Mixed vegetables (e.g., bell peppers, cucumbers)
- lemon-tahini dressing

Instructions:

1. Combine cooked chickpeas, quinoa, and mixed vegetables in a bowl.
2. Drizzle with lemon-tahini dressing.

3. Turkey and Avocado Wrap:

Ingredients:

- Sliced turkey breast
- Avocado slices

- Whole-grain tortilla
- Mixed greens
- light vinaigrette dressing

Instructions:

1. Layer sliced turkey, avocado, and mixed greens on a whole-grain tortilla.
2. Drizzle with a light vinaigrette dressing and wrap.

4. Lentil Soup:

Ingredients:

- Cooked lentils
- Mixed vegetables (e.g., carrots, celery, onions)
- Vegetable broth
- Seasonings (e.g., cumin, paprika)

Instructions:

1. Sauté mixed vegetables in a pot until softened.
2. Add cooked lentils, vegetable broth, and seasonings.
3. Simmer until flavors meld together.

5. Caprese Salad:

Ingredients:

- Fresh mozzarella cheese

- Tomatoes
- Fresh basil leaves
- Balsamic glaze
- Olive oil
- Salt and pepper

Instructions:

1. Slice fresh mozzarella cheese and tomatoes, and arrange with fresh basil leaves.
2. Drizzle with balsamic glaze and olive oil.
3. Season with salt and pepper.

6. Spinach and Feta Stuffed Chicken:

Ingredients:

- Chicken breast
- Spinach
- Feta cheese
- Olive oil
- Lemon juice
- Seasonings (e.g., garlic, oregano)

Instructions:

1. Butterfly the chicken breast and stuff it with spinach and feta cheese.
2. Drizzle with olive oil, lemon juice, and seasonings.

3. Bake until cooked through.

7. Tuna Salad Bowl:

Ingredients: Canned tuna

- Mixed greens
- Cherry tomatoes
- Olives
- light vinaigrette dressing

Instructions: Combine canned tuna, mixed greens, cherry tomatoes, and olives in a bowl.

- Drizzle with a light vinaigrette dressing.

8. Sushi Bowl:

Ingredients:

- Sushi rice
- Sliced avocado
- Cucumber slices
- Smoked salmon or tofu
- Soy sauce
- Sesame seeds

Instructions:

1. Layer sushi rice with sliced avocado, cucumber, and smoked salmon or tofu.

2. Drizzle with soy sauce and sprinkle with sesame seeds.

9. Chicken Shawarma Bowl:

Ingredients: Grilled chicken (or tofu)

- Hummus
- Tabbouleh salad
- Pita bread (optional)

Instructions:

1. Place grilled chicken or tofu on a bed of hummus.
2. Top with tabbouleh salad and serve with pita bread if desired.

10. Quinoa and Black Bean Salad:

Ingredients:

- Cooked quinoa
- Black beans
- Corn kernels
- Red onion
- Lime-cilantro dressing

Instructions:

1. Mix cooked quinoa, black beans, corn kernels, and diced red onion.

2. Drizzle with lime-cilantro dressing.

11. Greek Wrap:

Ingredients:

- Grilled chicken (or chickpeas for a vegetarian option)
- Whole-grain wrap
- Tzatziki sauce
- Tomatoes
- Cucumber
- Red onion
- Mixed greens

Instructions:

1. Layer grilled chicken (or chickpeas), tzatziki sauce, tomatoes, cucumber, red onion, and mixed greens on a whole-grain wrap.
2. Roll it up and enjoy.

12. Vegetarian Stir-Fry:

Ingredients:

- Mixed vegetables (e.g., bell peppers, broccoli, carrots)
- Tofu or tempeh
- Stir-fry sauce

- Brown rice

Instructions:

1. Sauté mixed vegetables and tofu or tempeh in a stir-fry sauce.
2. Serve over brown rice.

13. Spinach and Mushroom Quesadilla:

Ingredients: Whole-grain tortilla

- Spinach
- Mushrooms
- Cheese (optional)
- Olive oil
- Salt and pepper

Instructions:

1. Sauté spinach and mushrooms in olive oil until wilted.
2. Place the mixture and cheese (if desired) on half of the tortilla and fold it in half.
3. Cook on a skillet until both sides are golden.

14. Mediterranean Quinoa Salad:

Ingredients: Cooked quinoa

- Cherry tomatoes

- Cucumber
- Kalamata olives
- Feta cheese
- Lemon-oregano vinaigrette dressing

Instructions:

1. Mix cooked quinoa, cherry tomatoes, cucumber, Kalamata olives, and feta cheese.
2. Drizzle with lemon-oregano vinaigrette dressing.

15. Tofu and Vegetable Stir-Fry:

Ingredients:

- Tofu
- Mixed vegetables (e.g., bell peppers, broccoli, snap peas)
- Stir-fry sauce
- Brown rice or cauliflower rice

Instructions:

1. Sauté tofu and mixed vegetables in a stir-fry sauce.
2. Serve over brown rice or cauliflower rice.

Dinner

1. Baked Lemon Herb Chicken:

Ingredients:

- Chicken breasts
- Lemon juice
- Olive oil
- Garlic
- Fresh herbs (e.g., rosemary, thyme)
- Salt and pepper

Instructions:

1. Mix lemon juice, olive oil, garlic, and fresh herbs.
2. Marinate chicken breasts in the mixture.
3. Bake until cooked through.

2. Quinoa-Stuffed Bell Peppers:

- **Ingredients:** Bell peppers
- Cooked quinoa
- Ground turkey or black beans (for a vegetarian option)
- Diced tomatoes
- Onion
- Garlic
- Spices (e.g., cumin, chili powder)

Instructions:

1. Cut the tops off bell peppers and remove the seeds.
2. Mix cooked quinoa, ground turkey or black beans, diced tomatoes, onion, garlic, and spices.
3. Stuff the bell peppers and bake until tender.

3. Grilled Salmon with Asparagus:

Ingredients: Salmon fillets

- Fresh asparagus
- Olive oil
- Lemon zest
- Dill
- Salt and pepper

Instructions:

1. Season salmon with olive oil, lemon zest, dill, salt, and pepper.
2. Grill salmon and asparagus until cooked.

4. Lentil and Vegetable Curry:

Ingredients: Lentils

- Mixed vegetables (e.g., carrots, cauliflower, bell peppers)

- Coconut milk
- Curry spices (e.g., turmeric, cumin, coriander)

Instructions: Cook lentils and mixed vegetables in coconut milk with curry spices.

5. Cauliflower Fried Rice:

Ingredients: Cauliflower rice

- Shrimp or tofu
- Mixed vegetables (e.g., peas, carrots, bell peppers)
- Soy sauce
- Sesame oil
- Scrambled eggs (optional)

Instructions:

1. Sauté shrimp or tofu and mixed vegetables in sesame oil.
2. Add cauliflower rice and soy sauce.
3. Optionally, add scrambled eggs.

6. Baked Sweet Potato with Black Bean Salsa:

Ingredients: Sweet potatoes

- Black beans
- Diced tomatoes

- Red onion
- Cilantro
- Lime juice
- Avocado (optional)

Instructions:

1. Bake sweet potatoes until tender.
2. Mix black beans, diced tomatoes, red onion, cilantro, and lime juice.
3. Top sweet potatoes with black bean salsa and sliced avocado, if desired.

7. Teriyaki Chicken Stir-Fry:

Ingredients:

- Chicken breast or tofu
- Mixed vegetables (e.g., broccoli, bell peppers, snap peas)
- Teriyaki sauce
- Brown rice

Instructions:

1. Sauté chicken or tofu and mixed vegetables in teriyaki sauce.
2. Serve over brown rice.

8. Zucchini Noodles with Pesto:

Ingredients:

- Zucchini noodles (zoodles)
- Homemade or store-bought pesto
- Cherry tomatoes
- Pine nuts
- Parmesan cheese (optional)

Instructions:

1. Toss zucchini noodles with pesto.
2. Top with halved cherry tomatoes, pine nuts, and Parmesan cheese if desired.

9. Stuffed Portobello Mushrooms:

Ingredients:

- Portobello mushrooms
- Spinach
- Feta cheese
- Balsamic glaze
- Olive oil
- Garlic
- Salt and pepper

Instructions:

1. Sauté spinach and garlic in olive oil.
2. Stuff portobello mushrooms with spinach and feta cheese, and drizzle with balsamic glaze.
3. Bake until the mushrooms are tender.

10. Ratatouille:

Ingredients:

- Eggplant
- Zucchini
- Bell peppers
- Tomatoes
- Onion
- Garlic
- Olive oil
- Fresh herbs (e.g., basil, thyme)
- Salt and pepper

Instructions:

1. Layer sliced eggplant, zucchini, bell peppers, tomatoes, onion, and garlic.
2. Drizzle with olive oil and add fresh herbs, salt, and pepper.
3. Bake until the vegetables are tender.

11. Baked Cod with Tomato and Olive Salsa:

Ingredients: Cod fillets, Cherry tomatoes

- Kalamata olives
- Red onion
- Fresh basil
- Lemon juice
- Olive oil
- Salt and pepper

Instructions:

1. Mix cherry tomatoes, Kalamata olives, red onion, fresh basil, lemon juice, olive oil, salt, and pepper.
2. Top the cod fillets with the salsa and bake.

12. Turkey and Vegetable Stir-Fry:

Ingredients: Ground turkey

- Mixed vegetables (e.g., broccoli, carrots, bell peppers)
- Low-sodium stir-fry sauce
- Brown rice

Instructions:

1. Sauté ground turkey and mixed vegetables in a low-sodium stir-fry sauce.

2. Serve over brown rice.

13. Chicken and Vegetable Foil Packets:

Ingredients:

- Chicken breasts
- Mixed vegetables (e.g., zucchini, bell peppers, onions)
- Olive oil
- Seasonings (e.g., garlic powder, paprika)
- Lemon slices

Instructions:

1. Place chicken breasts and mixed vegetables on foil sheets.
2. Drizzle with olive oil, add seasonings, and add lemon slices.
3. Fold the foil into packets and bake until cooked.

14. Shrimp and Asparagus Stir-Fry:

Ingredients: Shrimp, Asparagus

- Garlic
- Ginger
- Soy sauce
- Sesame oil
- Red pepper flakes (optional)

- Brown rice

Instructions:

1. Sauté shrimp, asparagus, garlic, and ginger in a mixture of soy sauce, sesame oil, and red pepper flakes.
2. Serve over brown rice.

15. Butternut Squash and Chickpea Curry:

Ingredients: Butternut squash

- Chickpeas
- Coconut milk
- Curry spices (e.g., curry powder, turmeric, cayenne pepper)
- Spinach

Instructions:

1. Cook butternut squash and chickpeas in coconut milk with curry spices.
2. Add the spinach and simmer until wilted.

Snacks

1. Greek Yogurt with Berries:

Ingredients: Greek yogurt

- Mixed berries

- Honey (optional)

Instructions:

1. Scoop Greek yogurt into a bowl.
2. Top with mixed berries and drizzle with honey if desired.

2. Apple Slices with Almond Butter:

Ingredients: Apple slices and Almond butter

Instructions:

1. Spread almond butter on apple slices for a crunchy and creamy combo.

3. Hummus and Veggie Sticks:

Ingredients: Hummus, Carrot, cucumber, and bell pepper sticks

Instructions:

1. Dip veggie sticks into hummus for a satisfying snack.

4. Cottage Cheese with Pineapple:

Ingredients:

- Cottage cheese
- Pineapple chunks

Instructions:

1. Combine cottage cheese and pineapple chunks for a sweet and savory snack.

5. Avocado and Tomato Slices:

Ingredients:

- Avocado slices
- Tomato slices
- Salt and pepper

Instructions:

1. Season avocado and tomato slices with salt and pepper.

6. Mixed Nuts and Dried Fruits:

Ingredients:

- Mixed nuts (e.g., almonds, walnuts, cashews)
- Dried fruits (e.g., raisins, apricots, and cranberries)

Instructions:

1. Create your own trail mix by combining mixed nuts and dried fruits.

7. Hard-Boiled Eggs:

Ingredients:

- Hard-boiled eggs
- Salt and pepper

Instructions:

1. Sprinkle hard-boiled eggs with salt and pepper for a protein-packed snack.

8. Sliced Cucumber with Tuna:

Ingredients:

- Cucumber slices
- Canned tuna
- Olive oil
- Lemon juice
- Dill (optional)

Instructions:

1. Top cucumber slices with tuna, a drizzle of olive oil, lemon juice, and dill, if desired.

9. Popcorn with Nutritional Yeast:

Ingredients:

- Air-popped popcorn

- Nutritional yeast
- Seasonings (e.g., paprika, garlic powder)

Instructions:

1. Sprinkle air-popped popcorn with nutritional yeast and your favorite seasonings.

10. Edamame with Sea Salt:

Ingredients:

- Steamed edamame
- Sea salt

Instructions:

1. Sprinkle steamed edamame with sea salt for a savory and protein-rich snack.

11. Sliced Bell Peppers with Guacamole:

Ingredients:

- Bell pepper slices
- Homemade or store-bought guacamole

Instructions:

1. Dip bell pepper slices into guacamole for a tasty snack.

12. Greek Tzatziki Dip with Cucumber:

Ingredients:

- Greek yogurt
- Cucumber slices

Instructions:

1. Use Greek yogurt as a dip for fresh cucumber slices.

13. Rice Cakes with Almond Butter and Banana:

Ingredients:

- Rice cakes
- Almond butter
- Banana slices

Instructions:

1. Spread almond butter on rice cakes and top with banana slices.

14. Cherry Tomatoes with Mozzarella:

Ingredients:

- Cherry tomatoes
- Fresh mozzarella cheese
- Fresh basil leaves

- Balsamic glaze
- Olive oil
- Salt and pepper

Instructions:

1. Thread cherry tomatoes, mozzarella, and basil leaves on toothpicks.
2. Drizzle with balsamic glaze, olive oil, salt, and pepper.

15. Kale Chips:

Ingredients:

- Fresh kale leaves
- Olive oil
- Seasonings (e.g., garlic powder, paprika)

Instructions:

1. Toss kale leaves with olive oil and seasonings.
2. Bake until crispy to make your own kale chips.

CHAPTER FIVE

TRACKING PROGRESS

The Role of Monitoring in Weight Loss

In order to stay on track, make wise decisions, and eventually reach their weight reduction objectives, monitoring is vital to weight loss.

1. Accountability: The act of monitoring fosters a sense of responsibility. People are more likely to stick to their weight reduction goals and make healthier decisions when they keep track of their progress. Being aware of their accountability for their actions might spur people to persevere.

2. Awareness: Monitoring encourages people to reflect on their eating patterns, levels of exercise, and general lifestyle choices. It can expose trends and actions that might lead to weight gain, enabling the required corrections.

3. Setting the Goal: Individuals can set specific, measurable weight loss goals with regular monitoring. They remain focused and motivated by monitoring their progress toward these objectives. It also gives you a chance to rejoice in tiny accomplishments along the way.

4. Calorie Knowledge: People can have a better understanding of the connection between their diet and weight by keeping track of their food intake, portion sizes, and calorie intake. They gain the ability to make better decisions and successfully control their calorie intake.

5. Nutritional Balance: Monitoring calorie intake frequently results in a better understanding of nutritional balance. People may make sure they are obtaining the nutrients they need, managing their portion sizes, and limiting their intake of bad foods.

6. Physical Exercise: People can determine whether they are accomplishing their fitness goals by tracking their workout regimens and levels of physical activity. They can modify their exercises as necessary to enhance calorie burning and muscular growth.

7. Modification of behavior: Regular observation might help find the causes of overeating or harmful behaviors. People can work on altering their behavior and implementing healthier alternatives if they are aware of this.

8. Recommendations: Monitoring offers insightful input on the aspects of a weight loss strategy that are and are not functioning. People can examine their statistics to find areas for improvement and make the required adjustments if progress pauses.

9. Plateaus can be prevented by: With moments of rapid progress and plateaus, weight reduction frequently follows a non-linear pattern. By changing their food or exercise habits, people can use monitoring to identify and get past plateaus.

10. Monitoring: Monitoring can help with stress reduction, which is a factor in weight loss. Decisions are made based on evidence rather than uncertainty, which gives the process a sense of control and manageability.

11. Motivating factors: It can be very motivating to notice improvements over time, such as weight loss, increased fitness, or healthier eating patterns. It serves as confirmation that efforts are paying off and motivates people to keep up their weight loss efforts.

12. Long-Term Upkeep: Monitoring doesn't stop when you reach your goal weight. It is equally crucial to make sure people maintain their weight reduction progress and avoid gaining it back during the maintenance period.

Keeping a Food Journal

Keeping a food journal is an important tool for anyone trying to control their weight, change their eating patterns, or reach specific nutritional and health goals. You must keep track of everything you consume during the day.

1. Be honest: Keep a log of all your meals, snacks, drinks, and portion amounts. To accurately comprehend you're eating patterns, you must be honest.

2. Describe in detail: Not only should you record what you eat but also the time and place, how you were feeling, and any hunger or cravings you may have. These specifics can help shed light on your eating habits.

3. Use technology: Take into account using online resources or smartphone apps made specifically for tracking calorie consumption. They can facilitate the procedure and offer nutrient data for the items you log.

4. Calculate Portions: Use measuring cups, a food scale, or visual aids (such as a deck of cards for meat or a tennis ball for fruit) to precisely estimate portion sizes. This helps avoid estimating servings too small or too large.

5. Be consistent: Make an effort to log your snacks and meals at the same time each day. It is easier to spot patterns in your eating habits when you are consistent.

6. Include beverages: Don't forget to keep track of the beverages you consume because they might add to your daily calorie consumption, such as sugary drinks or excessive amounts of coffee with extra cream and sugar.

7. Regularly review: Regularly read through your food journal. Search for patterns, reasons why people overeat, or areas where they may get better.

Benefits of Maintaining a Food Journal:

1. Enhanced Awareness: Keeping a food journal helps you become more aware of your eating patterns. It assists you in locating potential problem eating areas or unhealthy dietary regions.

2. Responsibility: Maintaining a food diary fosters responsibility. Your decision-making improves as a result of your increased accountability for your actions.

3. Determining Patterns: By keeping a diary of your meals, you can spot trends in your eating habits. This can assist you in identifying the causes of emotional eating, overeating, or unhealthy snacking.

4. Goal Tracking: If you have certain dietary or weight loss objectives, a food journal enables you to monitor your development and modify your diet as necessary.

5. Portion control: It makes you more conscious of serving amounts and helps you avoid unintended overeating.

6. Nutritional Balance: A meal diary can reveal whether you're consuming a variety of macronutrients (carbohydrates, proteins, and fats) and micronutrients (vitamins and minerals) in a balanced manner.

7. Problem-Solving: A meal journal can be used as a tool to help you solve problems when you're eating habits or weight reduction journey face obstacles. The data can be analyzed to find areas that need improvement.

8. Motivating factors: Long-term improvements in your eating habits or weight can be helpful. It validates your efforts and motivates you to keep making better decisions.

9. Communication with Professionals: Keeping a food diary can help you and your healthcare professional, nutritionist, or dietitian have more fruitful conversations and provide more tailored advice.

Tracking Physical Activity

A healthy lifestyle must include tracking physical activity, which can be especially beneficial for those trying to lose weight, get fitter, or improve their overall fitness.

Guidelines for Monitoring Physical Activity

1. Select a tracking technique: There are numerous methods for keeping track of physical activity, including pedometers, fitness trackers, smartphone apps, and traditional pen and paper diaries. Choose a strategy that meets your preferences and requirements.

2. Establish Specific Goals: Set definite, attainable goals for your physical activity before you start tracking. Having defined goals will direct your tracking efforts, whether it's increasing daily steps, preparing for a marathon, or gaining muscle.

3. Consistency is important: Try to keep your tracking of your physical activities consistent. At the same time every day or following each session, log your exercises or other activities. This consistency aids in producing a trustworthy record of your advancement.

4. Record the Following Information: Include information about the type of exercise, its duration, its intensity (low, moderate, or high), and any other notes (such as how you felt during the workout) while keeping track of your physical activity. You can accurately evaluate your efforts with this information.

5. Utilize technology: Tracking physical activity is made easy by the features that many fitness apps and wearables offer. They can offer real-time information on heart rate, steps taken, distance traveled, and calories burned. These resources can be highly enlightening and motivating.

6. Include a range of physical activities in your tracking: such as sports, flexibility exercises, weight training, and cardio. This guarantees a well-rounded fitness regimen and keeps things interesting.

7. Set a reminder to: Create reminders or alerts on your smartphone or fitness tracker if you frequently forget to record your exercise. Tracking your development consistently is essential for accurately gauging it.

8. Monitor Development Over Time: Review your tracked data frequently to monitor your progress toward your objectives. Search for patterns, upgrades, or potential improvement areas.

The advantages of monitoring physical activity are:

1. Accountability: Tracking makes you responsible for achieving your fitness objectives. It motivates you to maintain consistency and drive.

2. Goal Accomplished: You can monitor your progress toward your fitness objectives and make the required changes to your exercise program or intensity by keeping track of your activity.

3. Motivating factors: It can be very motivating to see advancements and milestones in your tracked statistics. It strengthens your will to lead an active, healthy lifestyle.

4. Awareness: Tracking enables you to better understand your patterns of physical activity. It may draw attention to instances where you could stand up more often and sit less.

5. Health Observation: You can monitor your general health and fitness with regular tracking. Your endurance, muscle strength, flexibility, and cardiovascular fitness may all improve.

6. Avoiding Plateaus: By tracking your progress, you can spot potential peaks in your improvement and adjust your regimen to keep progressing.

7. Problem-Solving: Tracking can provide useful information for problem-solving if you run into difficulties with your fitness path. Your activity logs can be examined to spot potential problems and come up with fixes.

8. Data-Driven Decisions: Tracking offers information that can guide your training choices, such as varying the length, intensity, or variety of workouts to maximize outcomes.

9. Communication with Professionals: If you're working with a personal trainer or healthcare professional, sharing your tracked data can help with improved direction and individualized recommendations.

Using Technology and Apps

You may achieve your health and wellness objectives, such as weight loss, improved exercise, and general well-being, by using technology and apps.

1. Apps for tracking your exercise:

Fitness monitors: Your steps, heart rate, sleep patterns, and other factors can be tracked by wearable technology such as the Fitbit, Apple Watch, or Garmin. These gadgets frequently connect with specialized applications to deliver thorough information on your physical activity and health measurements.

Fitness Apps: You can monitor your dietary consumption, exercise habits, and weight loss progress using apps like MyFitnessPal, Lose It! and MyPlate by Livestrong. For your convenience, they offer calorie and nutritional information.

2. Apps for nutrition

Meal tracking: You may log your meals and snacks, calculate your caloric intake, and keep track of your macronutrients (carbs, proteins, and fats), vitamins, and minerals with the use of apps like Chronometer, Yazoo, or SparkPeople.

Recipe apps include: Apps like Yummly, Food Network Kitchen, and Tasty provide meal planning tools and healthy dish options. You can look up recipes that suit your dietary requirements and nutritional objectives.

Shopping: Apps like Any List or Out of Milk can help you efficiently organize your shopping outings, ensuring that you buy healthy goods and preventing impulse purchases.

3. Apps for mental health and meditation

Meditation and relaxation: Apps like Headspace, Calm, and Insight Timer provide tools for stress management and mental wellness, including guided meditation sessions, breathing exercises, and relaxation techniques.

Mental health assistance: Licensed therapists are accessible through websites like Talk space or Better Help for online counseling and assistance.

4. Apps for Hydration:

Apps to remind you to drink water The importance of staying hydrated cannot be overstated. You can track your daily water intake and receive reminders to drink more water throughout the day with the help of apps like WaterMinder and MyWater.

5. Sleep monitoring apps

Sleep monitors: Applications like Sleep Cycle, SleepScore, or Fitbit's sleep tracking feature can evaluate your sleeping habits, wake you up when you're in a lighter sleep phase, and offer suggestions on how to get better sleep.

Workout streaming services include:

Online courses include: You may watch a variety of exercise courses from the convenience of your home with services like Peloton, Beachbody On Demand, or Daily Burn. They frequently consist of several training styles and fitness levels.

Apps for social accountability and support:

Fitness Communities: Utilize apps like Fitocracy, MapMyFitness, or Strava to connect with friends, participate in challenges, and track your progress. A strong motivator can be social support.

8. Habit-Tracking Apps:

Habit Formation: Apps like Habitica or HabitBull can assist you in creating and monitoring healthy habits linked to your diet, exercise routine, sleep schedule, and other wellness objectives.

Apps for telemedicine and telehealth:

- **Virtual Medical Visits:** Health specialists are accessible through telemedicine apps like Doctor on Demand and Teladoc for remote consultations and medical guidance.

- Take into account the following advice when utilizing technology and apps for health and wellness:

- Pick apps that suit your unique preferences and ambitions.

- Check the privacy policies of your chosen applications to make sure they respect your privacy and are secure.

- Use apps as tools to aid your efforts, but keep in mind that they are not a substitute for expert medical advice or direction.

- Use these tools consistently to monitor progress and come to data-driven judgments.

- Be careful of your screen time and strike a balance between it and other healthy activities.

CHAPTER SIX

OVERCOMING PLATEAUS AND CHALLENGES

Dealing with Weight Loss Plateaus

Although they might be upsetting, weight loss plateaus are a normal part of the process of losing weight. They take place when your body adjusts to your present food and activity regimen, which results in a stall in your weight reduction progress. There are ways to overcome plateaus and keep pursuing your objectives, though.

1. Reconsider Your Caloric Requirements: Your calorie requirements could fluctuate as you lose weight. Consider recalculating your daily calorie intake to break through a plateau. To keep losing weight, you might need to gradually lower your calorie intake.

2. Diversify Your Exercise: Your body may have acclimated to your training regimen if you've been following it for some time. Try modifying your exercise regimen by adding new exercises, increasing the difficulty, or altering the length of your workouts. HIIT, or high-intensity interval training, is extremely potent.

3. Strength Training: Include strength training in your exercise regimen. Even when you're at rest, adding lean muscle can increase your metabolism and help you burn more calories.

4. Watch the portion sizes: Be mindful of portion amounts because they can quickly increase over time. Even if you're eating nutritious foods, check your portion sizes to make sure you're not overeating.

5. Track Everything: Keep tabs on your calorie consumption and exercise regimen. You might occasionally overestimate the number of calories you're burning or underestimate what you're eating. Any disparities can be found with the aid of accurate tracking.

6. Review Nutrient Balance: Verify that your diet contains a variety of nutrients and is balanced. Sometimes, a deficiency in key nutrients might slow your metabolism or prevent you from losing weight.

7. Boost Your Protein Intake: Protein is renowned for its capacity to increase metabolism and serve as a satiating agent. Think about eating fewer carbohydrates and fats while upping your protein consumption.

8. Remain hydrated: Dehydration can occasionally be confused with appetite. To avoid mindless munching, make sure you are drinking enough water throughout the day.

9. Sleep Enough: Your hormone levels and ability to control your appetite can be affected by sleep deprivation, which could result in weight gain or plateaus. Attempt to get 7-9 hours of restful sleep each night.

10. Control Stress: Stress can cause emotional eating, which can result in weight gain. Use stress-reduction strategies like yoga, meditation, or deep breathing exercises.

11. Remain patient and upbeat: Plaques are a natural component of the weight-loss process. Remain upbeat and constantly remind yourself of your accomplishments. It's crucial to keep a positive outlook.

12. Seek Professional Advice: Think about speaking with a qualified dietitian or other healthcare professional if you've tried a variety of tactics but are still unable to overcome the plateau. Based on your particular demands, they can offer tailored advice and suggest improvements.

Staying Motivated

Although it might be difficult, maintaining motivation during your weight-reduction or fitness journey is crucial for long-term success.

1. Establish definite, attainable goals:

Establish definite, quantifiable, and doable objectives. Instead of just trying to "lose weight," select a target weight or a fitness goal.

2. Subdivide goals into more manageable steps:

Break up your bigger ambitions into smaller, easier-to-achieve steps. You can feel a sense of success and maintain your motivation by completing these mini-goals.

3. Construct a vision board:

Make a vision board with pictures, sayings, and reminders of your objectives to help you visualize them. Put it in a place where you'll see it frequently.

4. Discover Your "Why":

Define the motivations behind your objectives. What inspires you to be in shape or lose weight? Knowing your "why" can help you stay focused, whether it be on enhancing your health, your energy, or your confidence.

5. Monitor Your Progress:

Record your progress in a journal or with apps, whether it's your weight, measurements, or level of fitness. It can be extremely inspiring to observe changes over time.

6. Honor accomplishments:

Rejoice in your accomplishments, no matter how modest. When you hit a milestone, treat yourself, but pick non-food rewards to keep on track with your objectives.

7. Maintain accountability:

Tell a friend, family member, or exercise partner about your objectives so they can help hold you accountable. If someone is watching, you're less inclined to skip an exercise or choose poorly.

8. Change Up Your Routine:

Monotony may result in boredom and a loss of drive. To keep things interesting, mix up your workouts, try out some new things, or switch up the location where you exercise.

9. Look for Inspiration:

Join online forums to gain inspiration and make connections with like-minded people; follow fitness influencers on social media; read success stories; or engage in other online activities.

10. Use encouraging self-talk.

Show yourself compassion and refrain from critical self-talk. Keep your attention on your successes and keep in mind that failures are a necessary part of the trip.

11. Create a Success Image:

Take a few seconds each day to see yourself accomplishing your goals. This motivation-boosting mental visualization might be used.

12. Establish a schedule:

Make healthy food and exercise a part of your everyday routine. It is easier to maintain consistency if it becomes a habit.

13. Seek Advice from a Professional:

To assist you in setting and achieving your objectives, think about working with a qualified nutritionist, a personal trainer, or a therapist. They can offer knowledgeable direction and assistance.

14. Create fresh challenges:

After achieving your initial objectives, set new challenges to maintain your motivation. This could be taking part in a race, picking up a new fitness ability, or experimenting with various exercises.

15. Be patient with yourself and kind to yourself.

Recognize that improvement takes time and that obstacles could appear along the road. Don't rush things, and try not to be too hard on yourself. Keep in mind that the trip is more important than the final destination.

16. Find Joy in the Process:

Pay attention to the advantages of eating well and exercising. Enjoy the flavors of wholesome foods, your favorite activities, your enhanced energy, and your overall sense of well-being.

17. Regularly revisit your objectives:

Regularly reevaluate your objectives and priorities. If necessary, modify your objectives so that they continue to reflect your wishes and situation at the time.

Managing Stress

Managing stress is important for general health and can help with your fitness and weight loss goals.

1. Determine stressors:

Be aware of the stressors in your life. You can create coping mechanisms that are specifically aimed at the stress triggers you are aware of.

2. Practice meditation and mindfulness:

Mindfulness and meditation approaches can support effective stress management, anxiety reduction, and present-moment awareness. Guided meditation sessions are available through apps like Headspace and Calm.

3. Deep Breathing Workouts:

Engage in deep breathing exercises to relax your body. Try the 4-7-8 breathing technique: inhale for four counts, hold for seven, and then let out eight.

4. Consistent Exercise:

Exercise is a great way to reduce stress. Make regular exercise a part of your routine to release endorphins, which are known to naturally improve mood.

5. Give sleep first priority:

Make sure you're getting enough good sleep, as not getting enough sleep can make stress levels rise. Create a calming nighttime routine and establish a regular sleep regimen.

6. Time management:

Stress can be decreased by time management skills. To prevent feeling overloaded, prioritize your chores, organize them, and divide them into manageable steps.

7. Social Support:

Make connections with loved ones for emotional support. It can be reassuring and enlightening to share your thoughts and feelings.

8. Healthy Eating:

A nutritious, well-balanced diet can improve your body's ability to handle stress. Limit your intake of processed foods, caffeine, and sugar, which can exacerbate the effects of stress.

9. Keep hydrated:

Stress symptoms might be made worse by dehydration. To stay hydrated, sip lots of water throughout the day.

10. Don't drink too much alcohol or coffee:

Drinking too much alcohol and caffeine can increase tension and anxiety. To help control your stress, moderate your consumption.

11. Practice saying no:

Try not to overcommit. To prevent more stress, learn to say no when you already have too much on your plate.

12. Work on your relaxation skills:

To decompress and lessen tension, try relaxation techniques like progressive muscle relaxation, aromatherapy, or warm baths.

13. Establish realistic goals.

Don't overextend yourself by trying for perfection; instead, set reasonable goals.

14. Seek Professional Assistance:

If stress persists and becomes unbearable, you might want to go to a therapist or counselor who focuses on stress management.

15. Take part in stress-reducing activities:

Engage in interest-driven pursuits, such as reading, painting, gardening, or music-making. These can offer relief from the stresses of everyday life.

16. Set screen time limits:

Spending too much time online, particularly on social media or news websites, might increase stress. Establish limits for your use of technology.

17. Practice Gratitude:

Remind yourself of your blessings on a regular basis. Keeping a positive attitude will help you feel less stressed.

18. Get Outside:

Whenever you can, spend time in the outdoors. Even a little stroll around a park can be relaxing.

19. Journaling:

Expressing your thoughts and feelings via writing can be a helpful approach to relieving tension and finding clarity.

20. Acquire stress-reduction skills:

Take into account signing up for stress-reduction classes or workshops that cover mindfulness, coping mechanisms, and relaxation techniques.

CHAPTER SEVEN

MAINTAINING YOUR SUCCESS

Transitioning to Maintenance Mode

An essential and perhaps difficult stage in your journey to wellness is switching from performance mode to maintenance mode once your fitness or weight loss goals have been attained.

1. Gradual Modifications:

Make modest changes to your food and workout routines as opposed to making drastic ones. Maintain a healthy diet while gradually increasing your caloric intake, and gradually change your exercise program to concentrate on maintaining your present level of fitness.

2. Monitor and modify:

Throughout the changeover, keep tabs on your food intake, exercise, and progress. This will enable you to spot changes in your weight and make the required corrections.

3. Establish a maintenance calorie target:

Determine how many calories you need to maintain your weight and activity level, or your maintenance caloric needs. For assistance, you can use online calculators or speak with a licensed dietician.

4. Continue to practice healthy habits:

Maintain the healthy routines you've established while trying to lose weight. This involves choosing wholesome foods, maintaining hydration, and engaging in regular exercise.

5. Pay attention to portion sizes:

To prevent inadvertent weight gain, continue to pay attention to portion amounts. Watch your portion sizes, both at home and when dining out.

6. Continual Check-Ins:

Plan frequent check-ins with yourself so you can evaluate your progress and make any necessary corrections. Body measurements or weigh-ins on a weekly or monthly basis could be used.

7. Put an emphasis on sustainable decisions:

Decide on foods and activities you can sustain over the long haul. Avoid unsustainable, excessive diets and fitness regimens.

8. Finding Your Balance:

Finding a balance that suits you is key to entering maintenance mode. Although weight swings are common, try to maintain a healthy range.

9. Rejoice in Your Success:

Set aside some time to recognize your successes and the wholesome routines you've established. When you attain goals, treat yourself to something other than food.

10. Keep Moving:

Keep adding physical activity to your regular routine. Exercise boosts general health in addition to aiding with weight maintenance.

11. Maintain your connection:

Remain in touch with the support group you've established during your weight loss journey. With friends, family, or online communities, discuss your objectives and difficulties.

12. Be Ready for Difficulties:

Recognize that maintaining your weight can be just as difficult as shedding it. Be ready for temporary setbacks and plateaus, but don't let them demotivate you.

13. Modify as required:

Do not become alarmed if you see weight gain or other indicators of regression. The ups and downs are common. Review your objectives, make any required modifications, and recommit to your healthy routines.

14. Mental health:

Be mindful of your mental health. A number of things, including stress and emotional eating, might affect your weight. Maintain your use of relaxation and self-care strategies.

15. Seek Advice from a Professional:

When switching to maintenance mode, think about working with a certified dietician or personal trainer. They can offer professional advice tailored to your needs.

Setting Long-Term Goals

Setting long-term objectives is an essential first step to making progress toward your fitness and weight loss goals. Long-term objectives provide people with direction, drive, and a sense of purpose.

1. Be Particular:

Clearly state your long-term objectives. Instead of stating a general objective like "lose weight," be more specific about how much weight you want to lose, your desired level of fitness, or other measurable results.

2. Make them measurable:

Quantifiable objectives will enable you to monitor your progress. Use specific measures, such as body fat percentage, weight loss, or fitness milestones.

3. Establish realistic objectives:

While setting ambitious long-term objectives is important, they should also be realistic given your current situation, available resources, and time frame. Unattainable ambitions can cause disappointment and frustration.

4. Establish a timeline:

Establish a reasonable timetable for accomplishing your long-term objectives. Think about what you can accomplish in a year, six months, or perhaps five years. Setting deadlines fosters a sense of dedication and urgency.

5. Breaking Them Down:

Break up your long-term objectives into smaller, easier-to-achieve milestones. These immediate objectives serve as stepping stones for achieving your long-term objectives.

6. Aligning with Values

Make sure your long-term objectives reflect your most important values and priorities. You're more likely to remain motivated and dedicated if your goals are consistent with your values.

7. Make them personal:

You should have a strong sense of purpose for your long-term objectives. Think about the importance of reaching these objectives and how they will enhance your life and wellbeing.

8. Create success visions:

Take some time to see yourself accomplishing your long-term objectives. This mental imagery can bolster your resolve and inspire you.

9. Put them in writing:

Document your long-term objectives. This helps you stay committed to accomplishing them by making them more real.

10. Create an action plan:

Describe the activities and actions needed to advance your long-term objectives. What precise adjustments to your diet, exercise regimen, or way of life are required?

11. Look for Accountability:

Talk about your long-term objectives with a friend, relative, or group of supporters. Accountability can both keep you on track and support you emotionally.

12. Monitor Progress:

Evaluate your advancement toward your long-term goals on a regular basis. Measurements, diaries, or other tracking techniques may be used in this.

13. Remain adaptable:

Be willing to change your long-term objectives if necessary. Life conditions are subject to change, so it's critical to modify your goals to keep them relevant and reachable.

14. Mark important milestones:

Recognize and appreciate your progress. Recognizing your accomplishments can increase motivation and strengthen your resolve, no matter how modest they may be.

15. Remain Committed:

Stay committed to your long-term objectives despite difficulties or failures. To succeed in the long run, you must be persistent and resilient.

16. Reconsider and Update:

As you advance, periodically examine and update your long-term objectives. As your priorities, circumstances, and objectives change, make adjustments to them.

Avoiding weight Regain

Even though it can be difficult to prevent weight gain after weight loss, it is possible with the appropriate techniques and attitude.

1. Develop sustainable habits:

Put more emphasis on forming long-term habits than quick cures. Select a healthy, balanced diet and an activity program that you can reasonably stick to.

2. Continue keeping an eye on your food intake:

Even after achieving your weight loss objectives, keep measuring your food intake. Regular monitoring will help you stay aware of what you eat and let you know if any harmful habits are beginning to creep in.

3. Keep Moving:

Keep up an active way of living. Regular exercise improves weight maintenance and has many positive health effects. Include a range of enjoyable physical activities in your schedule.

4. Set realistic objectives:

If you want to achieve even more progress, set attainable and enduring goals. Avoid difficult-to-maintain exercise or severe diet plans.

5. Experiment with Portion Control:

Maintain your attention to portion control. Even eating nutritious meals in excess can result in weight gain.

6. Take Care When Eating Out:

Exercise caution while ordering takeout or dining out. Restaurants frequently serve larger quantities and calorie-dense meals. Make wise decisions, such as requesting smaller servings or a side of dressing or sauce.

7. Plan your meals accordingly:

Making healthier decisions and avoiding impulsive, less nourishing choices can be aided by meal planning and preparation.

8. Give protein and fiber first priority:

A diet high in fiber and lean protein can make you feel full and satisfied and lower your risk of overeating.

9. Keep hydrated:

Sometimes, hunger and thirst can be confused. You can prevent mindless munching by getting enough water throughout the day.

10. Reduce stress:

Emotional eating and weight gain can result from stress. Continue using stress-reduction methods like yoga, meditation, or deep breathing exercises.

11. Get Quality Sleep:

Sleep deprivation can alter hunger hormones and cause weight gain. Attempt to get 7-9 hours of restful sleep each night.

12. Maintain contact:

Keep up your network of supporters. With family, loved ones, or a weight loss support group, discuss your objectives and difficulties. Their support can be quite beneficial.

13. Deal with Emotional Eating:

Recognize the situations that lead to emotional eating and learn constructive ways to deal with stress, grief, or boredom without turning to food.

14. Regular Check-Ins:

Regularly evaluate your weight and development. Early detection of weight regain enables you to take appropriate measures.

15. Be patient and tolerant:

Recognize that slight weight changes are common. If you indulge or have setbacks periodically, don't be too hard on yourself. Getting back to your healthy routines is crucial.

16. Seek Professional Assistance:

If you have trouble maintaining your weight, think about consulting with a certified dietitian or therapist who focuses on emotional eating and weight management.

Celebrating Your Achievements

No matter how big or small, celebrating your accomplishments is crucial for sustaining motivation, boosting confidence, and reinforcing constructive behavior.

1. Acknowledge and recognize:

Commend yourself for your accomplishments. Consider what you've accomplished and the effort that went into it for a moment.

2. Set benchmarks:

Divide your more ambitious objectives into more manageable stages. As you accomplish each goal, be sure to celebrate. You can stay motivated by participating in these little celebrations.

3. Give yourself a reward:

Take into account non-food rewards as a means to rejoice. Give yourself a treat, like a day at the spa, a new book, a night in with the family, or new gym gear.

4. Describe your success:

Inform your loved ones about your accomplishments. Their encouragement and uplifting comments can be tremendously inspiring.

5. Make a vision board:

Create a visual representation of your objectives and the benefits you'll experience when you reach them. An everyday reminder of your goals might be provided via a vision board.

6. Keep a Journey Journal:

To keep track of your progress, keep a notebook or utilize a fitness app. A strong incentive can come from realizing how far you've come.

7. Arrange a celebration event:

When you hit important milestones, think about organizing an exclusive event to commemorate the occasion. It may be a little get-together with close friends or a private journey you've always wanted to take.

8. Compliment yourself:

Talk to yourself with kind words and show yourself sympathy. Recognize your own perseverance and efforts while you celebrate your accomplishments.

9. Examine Your Development:

Consider how reaching your goals has benefited your personal development and wellbeing. Enjoy the improvements in your life.

10. Pay It Forward:

Take into account aiding those who might be traveling a similar path or giving back. Celebrate your successes by assisting others in achieving theirs.

11. Take a break:

A quick break or period of leisure might occasionally be a fruitful way to celebrate. It's a chance to refresh and acknowledge your efforts.

12. Capture the Moment:

Document your journey with pictures or a scrapbook. A great way to honor your accomplishments is to reflect on these experiences.

13. Set new objectives:

To maintain your momentum, set new goals after celebrating a success. Set new goals for yourself to keep improving and succeeding.

14. Be grateful for the journey:

Honor both the final destination and the journey itself. Often, the act of pursuing your goals is just as valuable as doing so.

15. Join in the festivities with others:

Share success celebrations with your team or supportive community. Share your accomplishments and motivate one another.

CONCLUSION

. In conclusion, your journey to fitness and weight loss is a transformational one that requires a blend of calculated actions and a long-term success-oriented mentality. Your route to improving health and well-being is diverse and includes everything from setting specific, attainable objectives to adopting sustainable habits and managing stress.

It's crucial to comprehend how nutrition, macronutrients, and micronutrients relate to weight loss. You get the ability to make knowledgeable nutritional decisions that support your objectives. Additionally, a crucial component of your journey is to be conscious of calories and portion control, whether through tracking or mindful eating.

Monitoring your weight, physical activity, and food intake is essential for maintaining your progress. To make this procedure simpler and learn more about your behaviors, you can use technology and apps.

Innovative strategies to boost your metabolism and get over plateaus include using metabolic confusion tactics like cycling calories, intermittent fasting, carb cycling, and high-intensity interval training. When used carefully and with the right instruction, these strategies can be productive.

Although it is frequently overlooked, getting enough sleep is crucial for your overall health, including your metabolism. As a metabolic confusion method, putting sleep first can result in more effective weight loss and better health benefits.

A balanced diet that contains a range of nutrients, macronutrients, and micronutrients is crucial when making meal plans. You can remain on track, enjoy your meals, and achieve your objectives by creating a weekly meal plan and including enticing, healthy recipes.

Setting long-term objectives is crucial, but it's also crucial to smoothly transition to maintenance mode. Finding balance, maintaining healthy behaviors, and preventing weight gain are all part of this period.

You can encourage your progress and keep a happy attitude by staying motivated, controlling your stress, and appreciating your victories along the way. Keep in mind that obstacles will arise along the way, but with tenacity and fortitude, you can keep going forward.

Your journey to fitness and weight loss is essentially a dynamic and empowering experience that encompasses personal growth, self-discovery, and a dedication to a better and happier life. You may accomplish your goals, sustain your progress, and take advantage of the long-lasting advantages of increased health and well-being by combining knowledge, techniques, and a supportive mentality. To become the best version of yourself, accept the journey, keep your vision clear, and remain committed.

Printed in Great Britain
by Amazon

39136504R00086